A NURSE'S GUIDE TO
Cancer Care

A NURSE'S GUIDE TO
Cancer Care

Brenda M. Nevidjon, RN, MSN
Chief Operating Officer
Duke University Hospital
Durham, North Carolina

Kevin W. Sowers, RN, MSN
Senior Associate Chief Operating Officer
Duke University Hospital
Durham, North Carolina

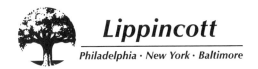
Lippincott
Philadelphia · New York · Baltimore

Acquisitions Editor: Susan Glover
Assistant Editor: Hilarie Surrena
Senior Project Editor: Tom Gibbons
Senior Production Manager: Helen Ewan
Production Coordinator: Michael Carcel
Art Director: Carolyn O'Brien
Indexer: Michael Ferreira
Interior Design: Melissa Olson
Manufacturing Manager: William Alberti

Library of Congress Cataloging in Publication Data

A nurse's guide to cancer care / [edited by] Brenda M. Nevidjon, Kevin W. Sowers.
    p. ; cm.
    Includes bibliographical references and index.
    ISBN 0–7817–1587–3 (alk. paper) ✓
    1. Cancer—Nursing. I. Nevidjon, Brenda. II. Sowers, Kevin W.
    [DNLM: 1. Neoplasms—nursing. 2. Oncologic Nursing. WY 156 N974 2000]
  RC266.N85 2000
                                 99–055266

9 8 7 6 5 4 3 2 1

We dedicate this book with great appreciation
to Jennie Simpson,
who kept this all together
with grace, dignity, and smiles.

BMN

KWS

Contributors

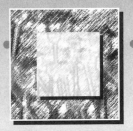

Elizabeth Abernathy, RN, MSN
Duke University Medical Center
Durham, North Carolina
*Chapter 14: Principles of Biotherapy and Gene
Therapy*

Laura Adams, BS
Duke University Medical Center
Durham, North Carolina
*Chapter 29: Changes in Cancer Care
Reimbursement*

Terry Ashby, RN, MSN, ANP
Senior Care Systems
Wilmington, North Carolina
*Chapter 22: Pain Assessment and Management in
People With Cancer*

Margaret M. Barclay, MSN, RN, CWOCN
University of Virginia Cancer Center
Charlottesville, Virginia
Chapter 11: Cancer Surgery

Cindi Bedell, RN, MSN, OCN
US Oncology
Dallas, Texas
Chapter 5: Breast Cancer
Chapter 16: Sexuality, Body Image, and Cancer

Susan Weiss Behrend, RN, MSN, AOCN
Fox Chase Cancer Center
Philadelphia, Pennsylvania
Chapter 6: Colon Cancer

Dawn Camp-Sorrell, RN, MSN, FNP, AOCN
University of Alabama at Birmingham Hospital
Birmingham, Alabama
Chapter 21: Constipation and Diarrhea

Terry Chamarro, RN, MN
Cedars-Sinai Medical Center
Los Angeles, California
Chapter 8: The Gynecologic Cancers

Mary Ann Crouch, RN, MSN
Duke University Medical Center
Durham, North Carolina
Chapter 9: Hematologic Cancers

JoAnn Dalton, EdD, RN, FAAN
University of North Carolina School of Nursing
Chapel Hill, North Carolina
*Chapter 22: Pain Assessment and Management
in People With Cancer*

Jeanne Erickson, RN, MSN, AOCN
University of Virginia Cancer Center
Charlottesville, Virginia
Chapter 25: Myelosuppression

Susan A. Ezzone, MSN, RN, CNP
Arthur G. James Cancer Hospital and Research
Institute
Ohio State University
Columbus, Ohio
Chapter 18: Nausea and Vomiting

Michelle R.V. Faber, RN, BSN, OCN
Duke University Medical Center
Durham, North Carolina
Chapter 19: Mucositis in Cancer Patients

Barbara Fristoe, MN, ARNP, AOCN
Virginia Mason Medical Center
Seattle, Washington
Chapter 15: Oncologic Emergencies

Tracey Gosselin, RN, MSN
Duke University Medical Center
Durham, North Carolina
Chapter 20: Anorexia

Rebecca Hawkins, MSN, ANP, AOCN
St. Mary Regional Cancer Center
Walla Walla, Washington
Chapter 21: Constipation and Diarrhea

Ryan Iwamoto, ARNP, MN, CS, AOCN
Virginia Mason Medical Center
Seattle, Washington
Chapter 4: Lung Cancer

Carla Jolley, ARNP, MN, CS, AOCN
Home Health Care Hospice of Whidbey General
   Hospital
Coupeville, Washington
Chapter 27: Dying

Wende Levy, RN, MS
Social and Scientific Systems
Rockville, Maryland
Chapter 2: Epidemiology of Cancer

Esther Muscari Lin, RN, MSN, AOCN
Chapter 17: Venous Access Devices

Molly Loney, MSN, OCN
MetroHealth Medical Center
Cleveland, Ohio
Chapter 1: Cancer Survivorship

Rosemary Mackey, RSCN, BA, MBA, FACHE
Mackey Krakoff, LLC, International Healthcare
   Consultants
Houston, Texas
*Chapter 31: The Challenges of Cultural Diversity
   in Patient Care*

Karen E. Maher, RN, MS, ANP, AOCN
Radiation Oncologists, PC
Legacy Portland Hospitals
Portland, Oregon
Chapter 13: Principles of Radiation Therapy

Lillian M. Nail, PhD, RN, FAAN
University of Utah College of Nursing
Salt Lake City, Utah
Chapter 24: Fatigue

Jill Nuckolls, RN, MSN
Duke University Medical Center
Durham, North Carolina
Chapter 28: Spirituality

Julie Painter, RNC, MSN, OCN
Community Hospitals Indianapolis
Indianapolis, Indiana
Chapter 12: Chemotherapy Administration

Sharon Pitz, RD, LDN
Duke University Medical Center
Durham, North Carolina
Chapter 20: Anorexia

Rosanne M. Radziewicz, MSN, RN, CS
MetroHealth Medical Center
Cleveland, Ohio
Chapter 1: Cancer Survivorship

Linda C. Russell, RN, FNP, MSN
Duke University Medical Center
Durham, North Carolina
Chapter 10: Skin Cancer

Jon Seskevich, RN, BSN, BA
Duke University Medical Center
Durham, North Carolina
Chapter 26: Complementary and Alternative
  Therapies for Cancer

Carol Sheridan, RN, MSN, AOCN
Golden's Bridge, New York
Chapter 30: Ethical Dimensions in Cancer Care

Gabriele Snyder, RN, MSN
Duke University Medical Center
Durham, North Carolina
Chapter 7: Prostate Cancer

Constance Visovsky, MSN, ACNP
Case Western Reserve University
Cleveland, Ohio
Chapter 3: Cancer Biology

Barbara Warren, RN, MSN
Hospice Palliative Care Program
White Rock/South Surrey
South Fraser Health Region
British Columbia, Canada
Chapter 23: Mood Alterations

M. Linda Workman, PhD, RN, FAAN
University of Cincinnati College of Nursing
Cincinnati, Ohio
Chapter 3: Cancer Biology

About the Editors

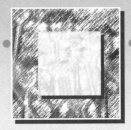

Brenda M. Nevidjon, RN, MSN, has served as Chief Operating Officer of Duke University Hospital in Durham, North Carolina, since 1996. Ms. Nevidjon's 25+-year-career in health care has included work in Switzerland, Canada, and Seattle, Washington, in addition to Duke University Hospital. She earned her BSN magna cum laude at Duke in 1972 and her Master of Science in Nursing at the University of North Carolina in 1978. She is a member of the inaugural class of the Robert Wood Johnson Executive Nurse Fellows Program and is a Johnson & Johnson/Wharton fellow. Ms. Nevidjon served as editor of the Oncology Nursing Society Newsletter for 10 years and has published extensively in the areas of nursing and health care, including her book *Building a Legacy . . . Voices of Oncology Nurses*. In 1995, she received the Duke University School of Nursing Distinguished Alumna Award. She serves on non-profit boards locally and nationally. She is married and has one son.

Kevin W. Sowers, RN, MSN, has served as the Senior Associate Chief Operating Officer at Duke University Hospital since 1997. Prior to his current position, he served in various leadership positions at Duke Hospital, having begun his career there as a staff nurse in a hematology/oncology unit. He earned his BSN in 1985 from Capital University in Columbus, Ohio, and his MSN from Duke University in 1989. He has lectured extensively on the issues of cancer care and HIV. Nationally, he has served on a variety of committees of the Oncology Nursing Society. He was the recipient of the Oncology Nursing Foundation/SuperGen Inc. Connie Henke Yarbro Excellence in Cancer Nursing Mentorship Award in 1999, and has been awarded the Oncology Nursing Society/Roche Laboratories Distinguished Service Award for 2000. Locally, he serves on the Duke University AIDS Research & Treatment Center Community Advisory Board.

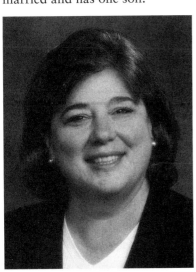

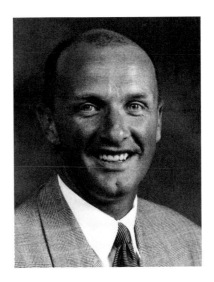

Preface

As we enter the new millennium, statistical projections show that cancer will become the number one cause of death in the United States. This escalation in the cancer incidence is occurring at a time when the rising cost of health care has challenged our current care delivery systems. Health care organizations have had to make many changes in the ways in which care is provided to people with cancer. During the 1990s, what traditionally had been inpatient care moved to the ambulatory and home setting. Across the country, hospitals, which once had dedicated oncology units, had to close those units and reintegrate the care of patients with cancer into general medical/surgical settings. We believed that there was a need for a resource directed to nurses in non-oncology settings who are caring for patients and families experiencing cancer. Thus, the idea for *A Nurse's Guide to Cancer Care* was born. As nurses whose careers have their foundations deep in oncology nursing, we have sought to develop a practical and affordable reference for nurses in hospitals, ambulatory settings, and the community who are dealing with the complexities of providing cancer care and education. We also believe that faculty and students will find this book useful, because most students will encounter patients with cancer during their education.

We designed this book not to be an oncology specialty book that encompasses everything about cancer care, but rather a resource to assist generalist nurses in understanding and responding to the clinical, psychosocial, and financial issues of cancer care. Clinical leaders in the specialty of oncology care have written each chapter, incorporating case studies, teaching information, and patient care tips to assist the reader to immediately apply new knowledge. The book is divided into three units to facilitate the reader's search for information.

In Unit 1, *Understanding Cancer*, chapters cover general information about the disease of cancer as well as specific cancers. The first chapter is about survivorship because we want the reader to know that people can and do survive and live full lives after a cancer diagnosis. We have included chapters on the more common cancers that we think nurses in non-specialty settings are likely to encounter. Content about early prevention, detection, diagnosis, and treatment regimens is addressed through each chapter on the major cancers. In Unit 2, *Helping Your Patients With Their Cancer Experience*, chapters focus on the frequent side effects of cancer and its treatments and how to help patients manage them. Side effects such as nausea and vomiting, hair loss, and pain are what people imagine when they hear the word cancer. The fear and anxiety associated with the word remain strong today even in the face of tremendous progress in diagnosis and treatment. Because the essence of nursing is caring and comforting, the contributors wrote these chapters to strengthen the reader's confidence in meeting the needs of patients with cancer. Unit 3, *Issues of Today and Tomorrow*, focuses on a few topics that are part of our world as nurses: the economic environment, managing ethical dilemmas, and providing care to diverse populations of patients.

The information inside the front and back covers provides the reader with useful references. Technology has made information readily available to the public, and patients are more knowledgeable than they ever have been. They often download information from various websites and bring that information with them. Thus we have included a comprehensive list of cancer-related websites. Also, there is a list of many national organizations and their toll-free numbers. Many of these organizations provide free or low-cost educational materials for patients. We encourage you to take advantage of these resources.

Many people made this book possible. Sue Glover, Senior Editor, understood our vision for a cancer care book for generalist nurses and was a great support to us throughout the project. We thank the editorial staff at Lippincott for their assistance in polishing the manuscript into the finished book. We would like to thank our contributors for their hard work in writing chapters filled with pragmatic information for their colleagues. We have special thanks for our assistant, Jennie Simpson, who kept all of us organized and handled hundreds of details.

In the next decade, as the healthcare world continues to change, one constant in the cancer experience will be a patient and family needing our care, whether or not our specialty is oncology nursing. Quality cancer care services will continue to evolve in our local communities, and each of us will have an opportunity to help shape their development. We thank you, the users of this text, for your professional and personal contributions to the lives of people experiencing cancer.

Brenda M. Nevidjon
Kevin W. Sowers

Contents

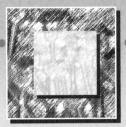

9   Hematologic Cancers   160
Mary Ann Crouch

UNIT 2

Helping Your Patients With Their Cancer Experience   271

UNIT 3

Issues of Today and Tomorrow   451

A NURSE'S GUIDE TO
Cancer Care

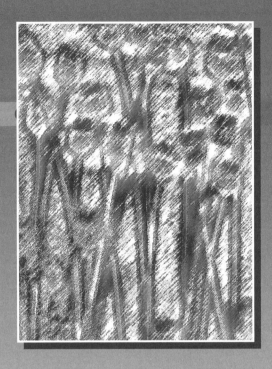

Understanding Cancer

Cancer Survivorship

CHAPTER 1

Molly Loney
Rosanne M. Radziewicz

According to the National Cancer Institute, approximately 12 million cases of cancer have been diagnosed since 1990. It is expected that approximately 1,300,000 new cases will be detected in the year 2000. With advances in technology, approximately 8 million people are living with cancer as either active disease or in remission (Abbey, 1997; American Cancer Society, 1999).

Although survivorship has been a theme in the literature for over 40 years, it is still an experience with many definitions and misunderstandings. Because survivorship can affect the individual and family living with cancer, as well as the community, it is important for nurses to have insight into what survivors face every day. The purpose of this chapter is to introduce nurses to cancer survivorship—as a lived experience, an ongoing and multidimensional process, and an important movement in society. Individual factors influencing adjustment in survivorship as well as nursing interventions for educating and supporting cancer survivors will also be discussed.

Cancer Survivorship: The Lived Experience

Mary had a busy week ahead, with two church events and three invitations from friends for dinner. She was very active for her 77 years of age and history of progressive arthritis. Mary didn't let a "little backache" limit her. Like her mother, Mary was always volunteering to help friends in need and to support community ac-

tivities. Maybe it was part of her Slovenian background that kept Mary focused on the welfare of others, instead of on her own aches and pains.

As Mary got out of bed Monday morning, she felt a new, sharp burning along her spine— so sudden and intense that it made her gasp for breath. She thought she needed to take her arthritis medicine for sure today. She had too much to do—John, a neighbor recovering from a stroke, was counting on her to help with grocery shopping, and Delores was—Mary's thoughts were interrupted by another stabbing bolt of pain that ricocheted like lightning from her middle back down to her toes. Almost in reflex, Mary laid back down and closed her eyes, hoping the pain would go away. But the pain stayed with her, and intensified each time she tried to get up. After an hour, her legs felt wooden and disconnected. She was afraid that she had somehow sprained her back yesterday while working in her garden.

After 3 hours of lying trapped in bed, Mary called her doctor. She was lucky to get an appointment for 1:00 that afternoon. It took Mary most of the rest of the morning just to get out of bed and into the bathroom to get dressed. Although her grooming habits were usually meticulous, today Mary could barely manage to wash her face. Mary was used to being the helper, so it was hard to ask someone for help. But now she had no choice. She called retired friends, George and Lucy, who said they would do anything for her, including drive her to her appointment.

By the time 1:00 came, Mary was sitting stiffly on the edge of a hard-back chair in her doctor's waiting room, in such pain that she thought she might faint. She was exhausted from the morning's struggle to move. She tried smiling to her friends, the secretary, the nurse, and the doctor, saying "everything is fine," but she was crying inside.

Two hours later, Mary was being admitted to the hospital for a diagnostic workup and pain control. A day later, Mary was confronted with the news that most adults in the United States fear. Her pain wasn't only from arthritis. Her MRI had shown a large tumor pressing on her spinal cord, causing pain and loss of sensation in her legs. Her doctor explained that if it wasn't removed surgically, she could become totally paralyzed and even die. Death wasn't foreign to Mary, but a tumor, and probably a diagnosis of cancer, were incomprehensible. How could she get sick? She had too many people and activities and flowers in her garden to tend to. Mary sat staring into the empty spaces of the hospital room, hearing the doctor's carefully chosen words, but feeling miles away—in a vast desert that offered no flowers or shade. Mary was numb, frightened, and all alone for the first time in her life.

How do Mary and other survivors begin to grasp what is ahead or what surviving cancer means? Mary's focus is on getting through the acute distress of pain, immobility, dependence, and fear—and on living through surgery so she can get back to normal. Although her doctor offers words of reassurance that people "can live with cancer," Mary remembers the many friends and family members who have died over the years after being diagnosed.

Thanks to early detection and effective treatment options, Mary's hopes for survival are promising. In the 1930s, few cancer patients had such hope. About one in four was still alive 5 years after diagnosis. Today, at least 50% of cancer patients survive beyond the 5-year mark. By the year 2000, it is estimated that survival rates will exceed 60% (Tuls-Halstead & Fernsler, 1994; Abbey, 1997).

Defining Cancer Survivorship

As people have lived longer with cancer, the nature of cancer survivorship has shifted. Historically, survivorship has been associated with living through

some catastrophic event, such as war or a natural disaster. But cancer, with its unpredictable course, is not limited to a single event. Traditionally, the American Cancer Society has defined survivorship as living 5 years or more after the cancer diagnosis (Breaden, 1997). Many physicians use words like remission and cure to represent survivorship, yet countless individuals with cancer continue to live with a partial remission or active disease. Defining cancer survivorship in terms of time or disease state does not give us the whole picture of living with the disease or the process of surviving (Leigh, 1998).

Although society still views cancer as a death sentence, cancer survivorship is a dynamic life-long process experienced when confronted with a life-threatening and life-challenging disease (Bushkin, 1995; Pelusi, 1997; Leigh, 1998). Bushkin (1995) described her experience as another dimension of living in the face of uncertainty, much like traveling along an unfamiliar road without maps or any sense of direction. Such a journey can be overwhelming, but Mullan (1985) views survivorship as a reason for celebration. It is the day-to-day struggle to live on, no matter what challenges develop from cancer or from life itself. Survivorship can become a victory in learning new skills and the resilience to live through, as well as beyond, the cancer experience (Leigh, Boyle, Loescher, & Hoffman, 1993).

What makes cancer survivorship unique is cancer's ongoing nature, treatment, and/or risk of recurrence. For many, the experience of cancer never ends. Like other chronic illnesses, cancer presents survivors not only with uncertainty but also with the need for managing new symptoms, frequent monitoring, accessing ongoing support, and trying to redefine self somewhere in between being ill and being well (Dow, 1990; Gorman, 1998). As a chronic illness, cancer has biopsychosocial consequences that can interfere with physical, psychological, and social functioning (Haberman, 1996; Leigh, Boyle, Loescher, & Hoffman, 1993). It can be difficult to discern how one level of functioning affects the other.

Stages of Survivorship

Mullan (1985) shared his own experience as both a cancer survivor and a physician in describing stages or "seasons" common to those living with cancer. Although general, these seasons can offer understanding of how cancer survivors move through their experience. His seasons include the acute, extended, and permanent changes (Table 1-1). Although each person will survive in his or her own style, the stages provide us with a reference point for assessment and support. The stages encountered depend on many factors, such as the individual's type and extent of cancer as well as response to treatment. After surgery, Mary will receive radiation therapy to control her cancer and prevent symptoms from returning. If successful, Mary's treatment will only offer her extended survival. With recurrence, she could quickly return to the acute stage, which would add to her cumulative uncertainty and fear. Survivorship involves many ups and downs, with movement between stages.

TABLE 1-1
STAGES OF CANCER SURVIVORSHIP

Stages or Season	Characteristics
Acute	• Begins with diagnosis • Involves extensive tests and starting treatment course • Focus is on meeting medical needs to contain the cancer • Survivor searches for information, acknowledgment, and ways to return to "normal"
Extended	• Begins when treatment ends, with maintenance treatment, or when cancer recurs • Focus is watching for signs of cancer and handling uncertainty • Survivor searches for ways to manage disease and treatment effects, such as body image changes, sexual dysfunction, and fatigue while regaining independence
Permanent	• Begins with remission or cure • Focus is on reentry into modified lifestyle • Survivor searches for resources in managing issues with employment, insurance, and long-term effects

(Adapted from Gorman 1998; Hassey-Dow, 1990; Leigh, 1998; and Mullan, 1985.)

The Experience of Survivorship: Issues and Nursing Interventions

Living with disease such as cancer affects the quality of life of the person experiencing the disease as well as those in relationships with him or her. In the last several years, quality of life has become more defined, studied, and used as an important measure of treatment outcome. In describing quality of life, there are common experiences that exist in each survivor's personal journey with cancer. Many propose benchmarks in the continuum of cancer as a framework for identifying the needs of survivors in adapting to cancer (Fiore, 1979; Mages & Mendelsohn, 1980; Mullan, 1985; Carter, 1989). Although it is important to recognize the benchmarks or phases of adaptation to cancer that most survivors may experience, current literature on survivorship is lacking in describing the process as a whole and the differences that make the experience unique for every individual (Breaden, 1997). The following themes in the literature describe the overall experience of survivorship. Although individual differences exist, this section will provide interventions to guide the nurse in supporting the cancer survivor and his or her family.

Issues of Self: Am I Still Whole? Who Am I Now?

With the diagnosis of cancer, the individual must learn to incorporate some new roles as a cancer survivor, a patient, a sick person, or a person who has limits into a new self-concept. Depending on his or her history, learning, and beliefs about self, this may be more difficult for some than with others. In a qualitative study about the impact of cancer on the perception of living in a body and living in time, Breaden (1997) identified the sense of wholeness that can be disrupted by cancer. Once treated for cancer, the survivor can experience an imprint that forever separates the sense of mind and body unity possessed before illness. A sense of discomfort can exist so that "even when one is 'cured' the experience of [cancer] leaves its imprint. Body and self are never the same again quite so comfortably united" (Pellegrino, 1982, p. 159).

Cancer can also cause a radical new view of the self that demands growth. Survivor stories focus on transformations that occur following the disease. Inner changes often center on a question of "what is to be learned from this experience that I must follow to stay healthy" or "who might I become now that I have survived." For some, this sense of surviving can be quieter, introspective, and less transformative. The way in which a person adapts to severe changes experienced in his or her lifetime is probably how he or she will experience survivorship. For others, choices are more marked and focus on new ways to live, to relate with others, or to maintain health.

Issues of Vulnerability and Fear: How Will I Make It? What If Cancer Returns?

Once the treatment occurs, the fear of recurrence is an ongoing theme for the person whose disease is considered not curable or is not surgically removed (Loescher, Clark, & Atwood, 1990). The body is perceived as vulnerable, and many survivors, even if cured or in remission, experience a fear that recurrence of cancer is never far away. The fear of recurrence can be expressed as overconcern or uneasiness to severe panic about benign symptoms such as minor aches and pains. Recurrence can symbolize an increased sense of vulnerability and sense of dread about the possibility of death, which can be a common reason for seeking psychotherapy for emotional distress.

Anxiety about recurrence can be heightened with the experience of aches and pains and can also occur at the time of routine medical visits. What the medical staff sees as a routine visit can be a major event for a survivor (Beyer, 1995). Patients mark their progress by the medical tests and checkups that are part of the treatment process.

Ferrel, Dow, Leigh, Ly, and Gulasekaram (1995) reported that psychological well-being is diminished as cancer survivors recalled their distress with the diagnosis and treatment. Fear of recurrence, secondary cancers, and metastasis contribute to this. From this information, the importance of developing teaching and support programs directed toward improving knowledge, dispelling myths, and providing understanding to counteract the fears is recommended.

Survivors can be taught to recognize the signs and symptoms of recurrence as well as new malignancies in order to prevent premature worrying about recurrence. Educating about self-examination techniques and setting up regular screening intervals and health maintenance exams can also allay anxiety about recurrence. The use of complementary therapies such as massage, relaxation, guided imagery and meditation, keeping a journal, and music therapy can be useful adjuncts to reduce stress and maintain wellness.

Issues About Suffering: Why Must I Suffer? What Purpose Does Suffering Hold for Me?

Suffering is a psychological experience when the sense of self is threatened. Suffering is also an evaluation of the significance and meaning of pain. The cancer diagnosis is associated by many with pain and discomfort. It is intensified by the lack of response by healthcare professionals to pain and frightening symptoms or in meeting psychosocial and spiritual needs (Ferrell, Dow, Leigh, Ly, & Gulasekaram, 1995).

The fear of suffering may be experienced as a patient becomes aware of others in the hospital or treatment setting with a similar diagnosis. Closely watching the deterioration and side effects of treatment may lead the survivor to consider such things as (1) "will this happen to me?" (2) "how much pain can I tolerate?" and (3) "what's the worst that can happen to me?"

One of the most important ways to counteract the fear of suffering is to begin to discuss the survivor's wishes regarding the management of disease and adverse reactions in the long term. Involving the patient in treatment choices and establishing open, honest communication also provides a sense of comfort and trust in the healthcare professional.

Issues About Treatment: What If the Treatment Does Not Cure Me?

The fear of treatment failure can direct a patient to seek information, establish nurturing relationships with healthcare providers, and risk treatment with the greatest potential for remission first. Uncertainty about the future is a primary concern early in the diagnosis that may be helped when options for management are provided. In the management phase of treatment, patients may still rely on the hope provided by healthcare providers for disease management or cure.

With disease progression, the patient may experience treatment failures. "Treatment failures force a patient to confront the 'realness' of the disease" (Ferrell & Dow, 1996, p. 34). The patient may experience more intense reactions than when first diagnosed since the hope for cure or remission is thought to diminish with each recurrence.

An approach of acceptance is recommended to reduce fear and anxiety. Mullan (1984) suggests that an expected and normal recovery issue is the fear of recurrence and treatment failure. Anticipating recurrence rather than cure helped reduce symptoms of depression, anxiety, and post-traumatic stress symptoms associated with recurrence (Cella, Mahon, & Donovan, 1990).

The term "failure" negatively affects the patient's feeling about self and his or her role in recovery, thus heightening a sense of vulnerability. In addition, these feelings occur with the patient having already experienced a multitude of side effects and anxiety with past treatment. Treatment failure results in questions about whether the survivor would again seek treatment, could tolerate the adverse reactions to treatment, or face the possibility of failure again. Listening to a patient's questions about personal endurance in future treatments is important in helping him or her make a well-informed choice about future goals and decisions.

Issues About the Future: What Does the Future Hold for Me?

Uncertainty about the future, progression of disease, and family responses to the stages of disease progression can contribute to psychological dis-

tress, fear, anger, and depression. Uncertainty also results in the survivor's need to exert control. This is a natural response to certain types of cancer that are not resected and are treated conventionally.

The ability to transcend the current experience and find peace in the moment is helpful during this time. Victor Frankl (1959), through his experience of surviving a concentration camp, described the ability of individuals to overcome difficult experiences and make meaning in their lives. Three ways were identified to accomplish this: (1) learning to give creatively to others, (2) learning to take from others by receptivity to others' care and appreciation of the world around them, and (3) learning to adopt an attitude of acceptance in situations that cannot be changed.

Managing the fear of uncertainty is important in adjusting to the disease, the treatment, the reaction of others to illness, and the family's experience. Some useful strategies to accomplish this include: (1) helping the survivor understand what is "normal" at various stages of disease progression; (2) discussing with the survivor what is and what is not within personal control; and (3) assessing the spiritual components of the survivor's life, which may identify strengthening supports in times of uncertainty. It is known that faith contributes to positive adjustment in life changes. This can be faith in oneself, in one's medical team, or in God.

Issues About Fitting In: Will I Ever Be Normal Again?

Joan, a 64-year-old woman, was diagnosed with Stage IV ovarian cancer. Prior to entering the hospital, she had been caring for her husband, who had Alzheimer's disease and a colostomy. She was concerned more about how her husband would be able to survive if she couldn't care for him. She has five adult children, but she also was worried about how the children could add the responsibility of caring for her husband. She wasn't supposed to get sick!

Part of adjusting to the diagnosis and issues of survivorship is learning to tolerate the side effects of treatment. For instance, fatigue induced by treatment or the diagnosis can contribute to a sense of not keeping up with the responsibilities of an important role, such as that of spouse or parent. Visible side effects of treatment, including hair loss and/or lymphedema, forces the survivor to face the world in a physical manner.

Discussion should occur on what the survivor identifies as goals and what are reasonable limitations within expected roles. It can be helpful to find a support network in which survivors can express feelings about the changes in their lives, where they desire to grow, and opportunities for growing experiences within the limitations imposed by their disease and treatment. It is important to discuss options so that the person with cancer can plan for the future as much as possible.

Issues of Control: Am I Going Crazy? Am I Losing Control?

Ed, a 57-year-old man, was admitted complaining of feeling tired and weak, with symptoms of the flu. After workup, he was diagnosed with acute leukemia (AML). Initially in treatment, he felt completely fine and would talk about his girlfriend's family, his enjoyment of porch visits with others, and the outdoors. It became clear to the staff that he was having difficulty dealing with treatment because it limited his ability to control his day-to-day life. Feeling trapped by the hospital room, Ed began to talk about feeling depressed and fearing that he would lose control, leave the hospital, and never come back. He limited visits from others and started interacting less and less.

The diagnosis and treatment of cancer challenges the survivor's sense of predictability and control. For some, illness can be the beginning of positive life changes. For others, it can be a time of despair. The need for control in treatment, family, career, and social life is important. In the initial stage of diagnosis, control can be obtained by deciding what is shared with friends and colleagues and at what time.

Suggestions for promoting a sense of control include:

- Discuss with the survivor what he or she chooses to share with the family. Help the survivor tell his or her story.
- Encourage the survivor to be an active participant in maintaining wellness (Beyer,

1995). Promote the philosophy that cancer and being healthy are compatible.

- Help the survivor make choices to promote a sense of wellness in treatment. Include nutrition and exercise in teaching about ways to promote a sense of control in treatment and disease management.
- Offer stress management techniques to provide a sense of control in a situation in which survivors perceive they are powerless. Techniques include relaxation and imagery to provide revitalization and control of symptoms; thought control over the fears, counterproductive thoughts, and feelings related to disease and treatment; and assertiveness to maintain control and self-worth in an environment of strong social pressures.

Issues of Guilt: Why Me? What Is It About Me That Is Letting Me Survive?

Waiting areas in clinics draw patients together, and they can share camaraderie and understanding of what each are experiencing. Support groups may also struggle with the loss of a member. The process of watching peers die from cancer can lead to many questions. Feelings of guilt about surviving while others are not—survivor's guilt—may be expressed. There may be mixed emotional reactions and many concerns expressed about the value of life.

Persons with cancer often feel the need to explain why they got the disease (Gotay, 1985; Shanfield, 1980). Explaining the cause of a traumatic experience can help decrease feelings of susceptibility to cancer recurrence (Loescher, Clark, & Atwood, 1990). In trying to determine a specific cause for the disease, previously unresolved issues may become questioned. Remorse for past wrongdoings or "God's will" can be used to explain why the disease was contracted (Bard & Dyk, 1956; Abrams & Finesigner, 1953).

Patients with cancer who have obtained positive meaning from the experience tend to have better adjustment (Taylor, 1983). Discussing the value of learning about positive ways to cope, living in a new and conscious way, and looking at life with fresh eyes and a renewed sense of values and priorities can be positive ways of finding meaning in the cancer experience that can replace guilt.

Issues of Unresolved Feelings: Why Am I Still Feeling Depressed When I Have Completed Therapy?

Indicators of effectively coping with a chronic illness such as cancer are a sense of hope, positive self-esteem, spiritual well-being, and the alleviation of uncomfortable mood states, such as anxiety and depression (Miller, 1985; Miller, 1992).

However, after the diagnosis and treatment of cancer, the sense of security about health and the environment can be permanently altered. Some survivors periodically report post-traumatic stress symptoms or recall flashbacks of intense emotion stimulated by a trigger reminding them of the trauma of cancer. Often this response is accompanied by feelings of intense sadness, hopelessness, and depression.

One might expect that there would be a sense of relief and joy on completion of therapy. What some define as remission can be identified by the survivor who is depressed as limbo (Leigh, 1998). An experienced mental health expert can promote adjustment in the survivor to mood shifts common to the cancer experience. The healthcare team may want to consider planning a "celebration of life" event for people who have completed their treatment course. Psychopharmacology, counseling, support group services, and other psychosocial interventions may be useful in promoting adjustment at the end of therapy for the disease and at any point during the cancer continuum.

Issues Related to Needing Others: Who Is There When Treatment Ends? How Do I Get Support Throughout My Illness?

When diagnosed with a chronic illness, patients are forced to walk hand-in-hand with the medical team. Once the treatment is finished, losing the vigilance of the healthcare team can be frightening.

One question that may arise is, "How do I get support when I'm ill?" Particularly if the patient has tended to be independent, the sense of needing others can be disturbing. In addition, dealing with the reactions of others to the diagnosis of cancer can result in additional feelings of isolation for the survivor.

Suggestions for promoting a sense of security about needing others include:

- Help the survivor understand the fear of cancer and the reactions of others to avoid feeling vulnerable.
- Help the survivor identify healthy relationships, which are major sources of support; this helps to strengthen the ability to cope and heal.
- Encourage the survivor to make self and health the first priority.
- Help the survivor to make plans for necessary changes in his or her role with family and friends.

Issues About Changing Roles and Relationships: Who Is in Charge? Does Anybody Really Care?

Social support influences adjustment to illness by increasing psychological well-being, improving treatment compliance, and reducing negative responses to illness (Lee, 1997). A supportive family and social network can lessen the devastation of cancer and clarify the important aspects of relationships during this time. During illness, a different kind of support and security may be necessary than when the survivor is feeling well and is most able to function. How well the support system adapts to this change determines in part how the survivor copes.

Helping the person with cancer with this issue can include:

- Teach the family about sharing roles and responsibilities during acute times so as to maximize family functioning.
- Recognize the need of the survivor or family to relinquish certain responsibilities and keep others in a flexible manner, depending on the impact of the treatment on the patient's ability to function.

- Help the survivor recognize the good intentions of friends and family. Accepting the help of others can ease the burdens and sense of inadequacy the survivor might feel.
- Help prepare the survivor for a variety of reactions from others, ranging from avoidance to full acceptance.

Personal Coping and Adjustment

A variety of coping skills are required to adjust to and live successfully with cancer. One's ability to cope affects how one perceives or appraises the situation, how well one relates to others, and how one can manage side effects of treatment, including pain. There is evidence that physical factors related to illness can be important determinants in the psychological adjustment of patients with cancer and that an "apathetic, given-up" attitude correlates with an earlier death (Davies, Quinlan, McKegney & Kimball, 1973).

According to Cohen and Lazarus (1983), people routinely examine what is happening to them; judge an event as either harmful, threatening, or challenging; then determine the degree to which they feel threatened or challenged. Based on their determination, people respond to the event or situation with coping strategies that they have developed in the past.

Studies have shown that patients who have the buffering traits of hardiness tend to adjust better and are less ill (Kobasa, 1979). Hardiness personality traits used to deal with stress include challenge, control, and commitment. "Hardy" individuals are thought to use this constellation of personality characteristics to differ in their perception of stress. Kobasa (1982) defined the characteristic of commitment as the ability to believe the "truth," providing a sense of purpose that diminishes the threat of a stressor. Control refers to the tendency to act as though one has influence on events and therefore tend to direct action on stressful events. Challenge is based on the belief that change is constant and that stress can be seen as an opportunity for growth rather than a threat to security.

Coping is defined by Folkman & Lazarus (1980) as "the cognitive and behavioral efforts made to master, tolerate, or reduce external and internal demands and conflicts among them" (p. 223). Coping skills are considered either effective or ineffective depending on their ability to relieve anxiety and reduce tension for the person involved.

Effective coping skills are those that, in similar past situations, successfully relieved anxiety and reduced tension. Weisman (1979) describes patients who cope effectively as being able to accept a diagnosis, seek more information, talk with others to relieve stress, and undertake some positive, constructive action.

Ineffective coping skills are defined by Ostchega & Jacob (1984) as those that:

- Stop the person from seeking treatment, interfere with treatment regimen, or foster noncompliance
- Cause more pain and distress than the treatment warrants
- Make the person give up everyday functions and usual sources of gratification, such as relationships with spouse/family and friends

Cohen and Lazarus (1983) identified several coping styles, which are described in Table 1-2.

Nursing interventions should be used to promote more effective coping strategies in dealing with the cancer experience. Some of these interventions can be targeted toward personality traits that the person with cancer possesses that will increase resilience to stress. Other interventions must be taught to promote effective adaptation to cancer. These interventions should include:

- Encouraging the patient to become an active and informed participant in the treatment plan
- Assisting the patient to look at the challenges of the disease and treatment more positively within the context of personal goals
- Helping the patient develop new coping strategies throughout the course of illness (being comfortable with a temporary lull in activity, etc.)
- Reinforcing social support, which can include family, friends, community and spiritual contacts, and so on

TABLE 1-2
COPING STYLES

Coping Style	Nursing Interventions	Coping Style	Nursing Interventions
Infomation Seeking: Gaining knowledge that has direct use in solving the current problem	• Give information needed at the time • Answer questions specifically • Repeat information • Ask survivor and family for verbal feedback • Individualize treatment plan • Provide written calendar with schedule of treatment • During treatment, provide blood counts as appropriate • Share medical information to clear up misconceptions • Encourage questioning and expression of feelings • Encourage use of supportive resources • Encourage survivor to remain as independent as possible	Avoidance and depression	• Encourage open expression of feelings • Assess activities that normally gave pleasure and include in plan of care • Involve in decisions regarding daily activities, treatment • Set up situations in which control can be exerted appropriately and independently • Guide in setting up short-term and realistic goals to avoid failure • Realistically offer reinforcement for completed activities • Involve mental health and social service in development of treatment plan • If survivor has lost or threatens to lose control, tell him or her you will offer protection
Direct Action: Doing anything physically or behaviorally to handle a stressful situation	• Encourage family to supplement survivor's self-care activities • Support family in how to be helpful with encouragement and reinforcement • Assist survivor/family in making decisions regarding treatment with the healthcare team	Anger and aggression	• Spend time assessing cause of anger, encourage expression of feelings • Recognize possible response to fear and not personalize • Be consistent in behavioral therapy • Reinforce attempts at assertiveness • Prepare survivor for tests, procedures • Involve family in all teaching • Reinforce family attachments through visiting or "rooming in" • Encourage decorating room like home • Encourage to ask for needed support • Encourage to use own support network
Intrapsychic Processes: What people say or think to themselves in order to gain control over feelings that might seem overwhelming to them Denial	• Spend time to establish trusting relationship • Listen for cues that mean the survivor wants to talk about his or her condition • Without reinforcing denial, talk in bits about reality; gradualy bring the survivor and family to accept reality at their own pace • Reinforce and support efforts to use other coping styles • Spend time with the family to discuss how to help the survivor cope	Turning to others: The survivor deals with stress through the support of others	• Spend time listening to needs and concerns • Encourage family support group and diversional activities

(Adapted from Cohen, F. & Lazarus, R.S. [1983]. Coping and adaptation in health and illness. In D. Mechanic [Ed]. *Handbook of health: Health care and the health professions.* New York: The Free Press.)

Factors Influencing Coping

Because cancer affects the individual and family as a whole, survivorship can become a series of crises or time of growth. Sudden and multiple losses of physical, psychological, and social function can threaten how basic needs are met and create stress. Ongoing and cumulative losses common to surviving cancer can drain coping skills and resources, which usually help to balance the negative effects of stress. Without these balancing factors, survivors and their families can become overwhelmed, victimized, and immobilized in coping with the process of surviving at any stage (Rickel, 1987; Loney, 1999; Van Fleet, 1998).

What factors influence or balance how survivors and their families cope? Several coping skills have already been discussed separately. However, it is important for nurses caring for cancer survivors to recognize how these skills or resources combine to strengthen coping, as well as how their absence can predict coping difficulties. Balancing factors can be categorized into the nature of the cancer, survivor characteristics, family characteristics, and support network characteristics (see Table 1-3 for specific factors).

If balancing factors are present, such as localized disease that is responsive to treatment, strong faith, an optimistic outlook, a supportive and flexible family, and a supportive church congregation, coping will be strengthened and crises will be resolved. In fact, building on past coping skills and developing new coping resources can help the survivor and family grow in their abilities to manage stress in the future (Aguilera, 1994). If balancing factors are lacking or are not used, survivorship can quickly become a time of crisis and further threaten survivors and their families with loss and uncertainty.

Survivor Characteristics

Characteristics of cancer survivors help determine an individual's coping style. Although survivorship is a universal experience, such characteristics as age, gender, culture, and past experience with stress can shape what meaning the experience has and how the individual and family respond to their experience (Anastasia & Carroll-Johnson, 1998). The following review offers some under-

TABLE 1-3 FACTORS INFLUENCING COPING WITH SURVIVORSHIP	
Nature of the cancer	• Type • Site • Age • Extent/stage • Response to treatment • Timing
Survivor characteristics	• Age and development • Gender • Education • Culture • Religion • Health beliefs • Personality traits • Past coping skills • Past experience with stress • Perceptions (meaning of cancer and of being a survivor) • Stage
Family characteristics	• Roles • Rules and traditions • Responsibilities • Communication pattern • Relationships with others • Past coping skills • Culture and values • Flexibility
Support network characteristics	• Availability • Culture • Accessibility • Past relationships with survivor and family • Range of services

(Adapted from Loney, M. [1999]. Loss, grief, and dying. In W.J. Phipps, J.K. Sands, & J.F. Marek [Eds.] *Medical surgical nursing* (6th ed.). St. Louis: Mosby.)

standing of how these factors can affect the quality of survivorship.

Age
• Cancer can occur at any age, although its incidence increases as people grow older.
• Losses surrounding cancer magnify other losses experienced in normal growth and development.
• When cancer occurs or recurs while the individual is trying to work through a developmental task, the accompanying stress can interfere with the individual's functioning and cause him or her to regress to an earlier stage of development.

- Cancer can impact on developmental crises for:
  - A child learning to control his or her body and the environment, exploring, and developing self assurance (Erikson, 1963)
  - An adolescent dealing with body changes, developing values, and relating with society
  - An adult struggling with starting a family, raising a family, or establishing a successful career
- Survivors may reenact developmental tasks that they have not successfully mastered or achieved at an earlier level (Daum & Collins, 1992).
- Cancer will be experienced differently at different ages or developmental stages, as needs and priorities change with age (Leigh, Boyle, Loescher, & Hoffman, 1993; Anastasia & Carroll-Johnson, 1998).

Gender
- The most common types of cancer include the following:
  - Men—prostate, lung, colorectal, and bladder
  - Women—breast, lung, colorectal, and uterine (American Cancer Society, 1999)
- Any cancer that affects sexual organs or function can threaten a man's or woman's sexual identity.
- Coping is learned through parents' role modeling during childhood.
- Men tend to have a problem-solving focus in coping, with avoidance of discussing feelings openly and an information-seeking approach to giving support.
- Women tend to have an emotional focus to coping, with open sharing of feelings and a nurturing approach to supporting others.
- Both men and women can perceive cancer as a threat and potential life crisis if it interferes with their gender identity and roles (Lazarus & Folkman, 1984; Predeger, 1996; Anastasia & Carroll-Johnson, 1998).

Culture
- African American men have a 20% greater incidence of cancer than Caucasian men.
- African Americans have the overall highest incidence and lowest 5-year survival rate of cancer, along with the highest mortality rate of any ethnic group in the United States (American Cancer Society, 1999).
- Barriers faced by minority groups help account for the discrepancy in statistics, including poor access to healthcare; inadequate healthcare services; limited knowledge about cancer and its treatment; fatalism over hope for a cure; poverty; ongoing life crises in meeting one's own or family needs; and distrust of healthcare systems.
- Culture is the "lens through which people filter and understand" life, as well as the cancer experience. Each culture has its own unique perception of the world and how its members fit in (Weekes, 1998, p. 62).
- Multicultural assessment focuses on the survivor, family, and their society within their own context of values, beliefs, and norms. It means looking into the influencing factors that can affect each survivor's experience without labeling or stereotyping (Varricchio, 1987).
- Survivors need guidance in understanding and negotiating the healthcare system as an unfamiliar culture of its own.

Past Experience with Stress
- Childhood cancer has a significant impact on adjustment as an adult.
- Cancer is traumatic beyond the diagnosis as the person is faced with treatment, isolation, fear of recurrence, and loss of body parts and function.
- Risk is present for post-traumatic stress disorder (PTSD).
- PTSD is an anxiety disorder with the survivor reexperiencing the trauma, becoming aroused when the trauma comes to mind, and wishing to avoid reliving the trauma (APA, 1994).
- Predictors to PTSD can include how frightening treatment was for the survivor, his or her general anxiety, the amount of time since the end of treatment, and family perception of trauma (Stuber, Kazak, Meeske, Barakat, Gurthrie, Garnier, Pynoos, & Meadows, 1997).

Family Characteristics

Each loss felt by the survivor can echo within the family throughout the cancer experience. Any change in one member will affect the other members, as well as the family function as a unit. Families usually try to maintain the way things were before cancer, by shifting responsibilities and roles to fill in for the survivor, but the ongoing stress that accompanies cancer can eventually exhaust family coping resources. Confusion can develop over who is responsible for what roles and what rules need to be followed. Families with conflict before the cancer diagnosis can become fragmented, and communication between members can break down at a time when family support is needed. Often, the stress can either help pull family members together or trigger family crises (Aguilera, 1994). How families adapt to the cancer experience is determined by several family characteristics (see Table 1-3). How the survivor copes is directly influenced by the family's flexibility in coping with its own experience (Loney, 1999).

Support Network Characteristics

A network of supportive relationships with family, friends, neighbors, coworkers, and community groups can help survivors manage the ups and downs of their experience. Active support not only promotes coping but also feelings of well-being and quality of life (Halstead & Fernsler, 1994; Raines, 1999). Social support helps to meet basic needs for love and belonging, self-esteem, and control while balancing stress to avoid potential crisis (Aguilera, 1994). Factors that influence support networks are listed in Table 1-3.

Social support can offer benefits to both cancer survivors and their families. Simply talking with someone who understands and is willing to listen can be reassuring for survivors who fear social isolation (Raines, 1999). Sharing experiences, fears, hopes, and achievements with another survivor can help normalize the survivorship experience, offer education about coping skills, and help survivors feel less alone. Research has found that women with advanced breast cancer lived 18 months longer by participating in a breast cancer support group (Spiegel, 1993).

Family members can also use peer support to better understand the cancer experience and find ways to tangibly help the survivor. Families often need help with raising children, meals, transportation, household maintenance, and babysitting. Friends, neighbors, and church groups can step in and offer specific help if their ties with the family are strong and culturally accepted. If support can reinforce the family in meeting its needs, the family can then offer more support to the survivor (Rendle, 1997).

Nurses can offer critical guidance to cancer survivors and their families in mobilizing balancing factors or coping skills by:

1. Being fully present to hear their story and build trusting relationships that convey "I'm here with you" (Osterman & Schwartz-Barcott, 1996)
2. Encouraging them to share what living with cancer means to them
3. Acknowledging losses
4. Helping them identify past coping skills and resources that have worked
5. Focusing on recognizing what skills and resources they can use to cope with the present
6. Helping them problem-solve ways to use past skills and resources, or develop new ones, to meet their needs and manage the ongoing stress
7. Reinforcing their abilities to regain some control

The goal of crisis intervention is to provide survivors and their families with the education, compassion, empathy, and support needed to develop or reinforce helpful coping skills, which can be used throughout all their seasons of survival (Van Fleet, 1998).

Physical Well-Being

The cancer experience challenges survivors not only with universal fears but also with physical complications that can occur during, and can continue long after, the diagnosis and treatment course. Many of these bodily symptoms contribute to the fear, loss of control, and emotional/spiritual issues facing survivors. A major component of physical well-being for the person with cancer during treatment appears to be symptom control. Several symptoms have been identified as having an impact on physical well-being, including dysphagia, appetite disturbances, taste disturbances, nausea, vomiting, constipation, diarrhea, sore mouth, dyspnea, fatigue, insomnia, changes in level of strength, numbness, and pain (Padilla, Ferrell, & Grant, 1990; Ferrell, Grant, & Padilla, 1991). Molassiotis, Van Den Akker, Milligan, and Goldman (1997), in a study of bone marrow transplant patients, found that symptom distress was a good indicator of long-term prognosis.

Despite successful treatment, many serious long-term effects of treatment can be discovered, sometimes decades after treatment (Hawkins & Stevens, 1996). Table 1-4 describes some of the clinical observations of long-term impairments related to treatment.

Identifying, monitoring, and managing symptoms during treatment can affect adjustment and promote a concept of wellness despite the cancer diagnosis. Surveillance after treatment ends is just as important in helping the survivor cope with long-term effects and worrying about recurrence. Survivors need ongoing opportunities to monitor, interpret, and manage symptoms. They also need education about what to expect through all stages of their experience (Johnson & Johnson, 1998; Leigh, 1998).

TABLE 1-4

CHRONIC, DELAYED AND POSSIBLE LONG-TERM EFFECTS OF CANCER TREATMENT

Effect	Example
Chronic or Long-Term Effects	
• Compromised immune system	• Increased infections, decreased immune function response
	• Pain, neuropathies, fatigue
• Functional changes	• Abnormal growth and final adult height
• Cosmetic changes	• Limb or spinal asymmetry
	• Alopecia
	• Amputations, ostomies, scars
Delayed Effects—Organ or System Failure	
• Reproductive	• Fertility problems, early menopause, reduced number of livebirths
	• Early onset of puberty
	• Breast hypoplasia and failure to lactate
• Endocrine	• Hypothyroidism from patients receiving radiotherapy bordering on thyroid
• Cardiac	• Abnormal cardiac function, coronary artery disease, cardiomyopathy, pericardial effusion, myocardial infarction, pericarditis, ECG changes, decreased LVEF
• Pulmonary	• Fibrosis, obliteration of alveolar structure, pneumonitis, loss of lung volume, veno-occlusive disease

Effect	Example
• Renal/ Genitourinary	• Compensatory hyptertrophy of remaining kidney following nephrectomy, nephritis, bladder fibrosis, hemorrhagic cystitis
• Neurological	• Decreasing attention span and cognitive skills, leukoencephalopathy
• Gastrointestinal/ Hepatic	• Risk of adhesions, hepatic fibrosis, and portal hypertension
• Musculoskeletal	Osteoporosis, avascular necrosis of bone, scoliosis, limb growth
• Dermatological	• Discomfort, excoriation, skin dryness, abnormal pigmentation, dermatitis
Delayed Effects From Treatment	
• Recurrence of primary cancer	
• Second cancers	• Bone cancer following radiotherapy to bone for childhood cancer
	• Leukemia for children exposed to alkylating agents, exposure to epipodophyllotoxins
	• Breast cancer following radiotherapy for Hodgkin's disease
Functional Problems	• Lymphedema
	• Hearing Loss
	• Cataracts, dry eyes
	• Reduced salivation
	• Disrupted dental development, increased dental caries
	• Tear duct fibrosis
	• Avascular necrosis

(Adapted from Hawkins & Stevens, 1996; Leigh, 1998; Hollen & Hobbie, 1995.)

Spiritual Well-Being

Spiritual issues affect one's adjustment to illness. For the purpose of this chapter, spiritual well-being denotes the degree of harmonious relationships with others and one's higher being. It can affect how one copes with the diagnosis and progression of cancer as well as provide a sense of purpose and meaning in life, help in preparation for death, and serve as a source of personal self-esteem (Hulme, 1986; Moberg, 1980). Through spirituality, a person can learn to overcome difficulties and live life more fully. Hope is often connected with one's spirituality. Fehring, Miller, and Shaw (1997) showed that in elderly subjects with cancer, there was a positive relationship between spiritual well-being and hope and positive mood states and a negative relationship with depression.

"Enspiriting" the Survivor

Archer-Copp and Dixon-Copp (1993) identified several nursing interventions that support spiritual nurturing of persons with cancer. These include:

- Giving encouragement
- Being quietly, professionally confident
- Demonstrating genuine respect for the survivor and his or her positive efforts
- Remembering to add personal touches to caring, recognizing special characteristics of the survivor
- Trusting the wisdom of struggling, standing by through the experience, and protecting space and privacy
- Being natural and resisting the temptation to be grim
- Helping survivors talk about their feelings

Helping in the Search for Personal Meaning

When faced with the diagnosis of cancer and treatment, many survivors struggle with questions for which there are few answers. Trying to find a reason for illness can be comforting and can signify a relationship between response to illness and one's spirituality. Questions such as these are difficult to share with others and are often unspoken: "What was my life like that resulted in the disease?" "Why me?" "Why do unfair things happen to just people?" Taylor, Lichtman, and Wood (1984) found that the search for meaning was an integral component to the cognitive adaptation to cancer. Many women, although not all, were found to attribute a positive meaning to their cancer experience. The experience helped some women with breast cancer readdress their lives, change their attitudes toward life, increase their knowledge and desire to change, and reprioritize their values. With new realizations, there can be a confrontation of the barriers to maintaining a healthier lifestyle. Some effort toward turning inward and learning from the cancer experience was a common theme in the majority of subjects asked about their personal experience (O'Conner, Wicker, & Germino, 1990).

Nurses are often faced with the challenge of staying silent or assisting in finding the answer to difficult questions about the meaning of the cancer experience. Johnston-Taylor (1993) suggests the following nursing interventions toward caring for the spiritual dimension:

- Assess patients with severe symptom distress, chronic illness, and those who are single, young, or who appear with adjustment difficulties.
- Be alert to verbal and nonverbal cues to recognize personal struggles in finding meaning for the cancer experience.
- Ask open-ended questions to elicit clarity and direction (e.g., "Have you thought of any possible answers to the questions you just asked?" "Do you ever question why or why not?" "Has anything good come from your experience?").
- Identify whether or not the patient is searching for meaning or simply not concerned about finding meaning with the experience.
- Provide active listening and insightful questioning; allow storytelling; and provide compassionate presence to facilitate discovery.
- If the patient desires, refer him or her to a chaplain or psychotherapist.

Inspiring Hope

Offering hope to cancer survivors can seem challenging, but the possibility for hope always exists. Nurses cannot "give" survivors hope, but they can:

- Communicate grounds or reasons for hope in the nurse–patient relationship (Koopmeiners, Post-White, Gutnecht, Ceransky, Nickelsen, Drew, Mackey, & Kreitzer, 1997)
- Be present by giving the survivor time to talk about whatever is on his or her mind
- Provide information with sensitivity about how it meets the survivor's and family's needs
- Show recognition of the survivor as a special person through expressions of caring
- Help the survivor redefine his or her hopes by setting short-term goals for each day, starting with today. Encourage focusing on the small activities, tasks, and interactions that the survivor enjoys rather than the global hope for a "cure" (Hickey, 1986).
- Guide the survivor and family in thinking about possibilities instead of limitations, no matter what stage of survivorship they are experiencing
- Encourage problem-solving of ways to make possibilities happen and achieve goals for the survivor and family
- Acknowledge the survivor's and family's goals and offer reinforcement when they are achieved

Issues With Cancer in Society

Persons living with cancer can face issues of employment discrimination, insurability, and financial support. These issues are often taken for granted, but they are important because they affect the survivor's general well-being.

Economic

With increasing demand for cancer care, hospitals are developing competitive programs to meet the rising demand cost-effectively. Costs are high due to increased inciddence of cancer in socioeconomi-

cally disadvantaged populations, high acuity care needs, the need for intensive monitoring during treatment, the growth of high technology, and the increased need for psychological services (Fleck, 1993).

Insurability

Many cancer survivors are experiencing longer lifespans after receiving treatment. Barriers to available adequate health insurance include refusal of applications, policy cancellations or reductions, increased premiums, waived or excluded preexisting conditions, and extended waiting periods (Hoffman, 1990; Crothers, 1987).

Because there are no federally mandated regulations on the provision of health insurance, survivors must examine the specific terms of their policies and be aware of state law to determine if there is a violation. State insurance commissions regulate insurance rates, policy conditions, and aspects of coverage and benefits. Questions can be directed to these state agencies. In addition, in some states high-risk pools exist to allow the purchase of comprehensive insurance plans. On a local level, insurance departments, the Social Security office, and local survivor organizations can be helpful in addressing concerns.

Employment Discrimination

There is insufficient literature to accurately report the frequency with which survivors experience difficulties with employment (Abbey, 1997). However, survivors report having difficulty at work due to medical problems (Hoffman, 1989), the impact of treatment (Dow, Ferrell, & Anello, 1997), and negative attitudes (Feldman, 1987). In addition, some employers erect barriers to survivors' job opportunities that may be illegal (Hoffman, 1997). Survivors can experience "job lock," or the inability to leave a job due to the risk of losing insurance, pension, or other benefits.

The Americans with Disabilities Act (ADA) can prohibit some types of job discrimination by employers, employment agencies, and labor unions against persons with cancer under certain circumstances and within the definitions of the law (Hoffman, 1997). The Act also provides for reasonable accommodation for medical appointments and treatment, prevents discrimination against families of cancer survivors, and assures fairness in the provision of health insurance.

Survivors can best avoid discrimination by maintaining privacy about their diagnosis unless it would affect job qualifications, by staying informed of their legal rights, and by requesting information about benefits after receiving a job offer and legitimizing their ability to perform the job. If suspicions exist about differential treatment because of the diagnosis, survivors should resolve employment issues using the appropriate agency's policies and procedures, focus on educating supervisors and coworkers, and suggest reasonable job accommodations. If efforts fail, survivors should keep accurate written records of all relevant events at work, evaluate long-term goals, and maintain their right to legal counsel.

Other Strategies for Helping Survivors Along Their Journey

Connecting With Support

Nurses caring for cancer survivors can play an important role in connecting with the person behind the cancer diagnosis and supporting him or her throughout the survivorship experience. Nurses can offer direct support through their caring presence, developing a therapeutic nurse–patient relationship, acknowledging the survivor's experience as it changes, educating the survivor and family about ways to meet their ongoing needs, showing respect for and sensitivity to the survivor's family and cultural practices, and linking the survivor and family to a variety of cancer-specific supports.

Cancer survivors and their families need information and encouragement in accessing programs that can help them cope with cancer as well as become partners in their health care (Johnson & Johnson, 1998). Psychosocial support programs can provide opportunities to release feelings and work through grief, begin to find some meaning out of the experience, obtain validation, share fears and concerns, and regain a sense of control in actively seeking information (Johnson & Johnson, 1998; Loney, 1999).

Because the needs and coping styles of survivors and their families vary, it is important to provide information about a variety of support programs. See the inside covers for a listing of available programs and resources.

Advocacy

With the advances in cancer detection and treatment, more survivors are living healthy and productive lives. A survivorship movement began in the 1980s and has gained momentum with consumer groups in the 1990s. The whole focus on "survivorship" has replaced the label of "victim" and the social stigma associated with cancer. Clark and Stovall (1996) recognized that successful adaptation is based on learning advocacy skills that can be used throughout the cancer continuum. These skills include:

- Learning to ask questions, get answers, gather and sort data, and access resources
- Communicating with the healthcare team as an active decision maker and self-advocate
- Developing problem-solving skills to help critique and discover new ways of handling difficult problems and conflicts
- Negotiating skills to help obtain necessary training, legal support, and employment opportunities and to deal with conflicts that may arise during treatment

Advocacy efforts can be useful in several arenas. First, on a personal level, being an advocate for oneself is a way of taking control in an otherwise confusing system of diagnoses and treatments. Being an advocate for oneself means being able to ask questions, obtain second opinions, locate resources for obtaining support, and arming oneself with valid information. These skills can promote a positive sense of quality of life in the individual.

Once able to advocate for themselves, survivors may choose to find opportunities to share with others in some meaningful way of "giving back." The survivor can advocate with a larger group, including other survivors, healthcare providers, or those in the political environment. These efforts may have a broader impact on survivorship movements.

Finally, advocacy may extend into the public arena. Affecting a change in public policy, participating in research, giving witness to survivorship, and contributing to the greater good can maximize quality of life on a personal and community level. Helping survivors find ways of helping others and finding a "cause" can be a way of empowering persons with cancer to live beyond their disease.

Thriving Beyond Survivorship

Although many survivors focus on just wanting to "get through" their experience with cancer, others find that survivorship is a time to thrive. Thriving involves becoming an active partner in the family, community, and healthcare system in searching for wellness—even in the face of cancer. It means defining oneself as a unique and talented individual, rather than as someone with cancer (Dow, 1990). Thriving involves understanding that having cancer and being healthy can happen at the same time. Thriving means a focus on the positive in any situation, instead of worrying about uncertain fears and signs of cancer (Beyer, 1995).

Thriving does not necessarily mean living longer, but living better in making the most of the moment. Cancer places the meaning of life and death in a new perspective. Individual and family values become clearer, priorities are directed more to personal growth, and faith is renewed. The experience of surviving empowers the person with cancer to take control and become whatever he or she wants to be. Even physical effects of cancer or its treatment do not stop a survivor who has reached this point from thriving (Dow, 1990).

Thriving is a subtle process that occurs over time, with much sorting of experiences and searching for some meaning. It can serve as a coping resource, although it is difficult to identify from the outside. Survivors who are thriving look for opportunities to tell their stories, with themes such as "Cancer wasn't the worst thing that happened to me," "Cancer was in my body once, but it's never getting into my neighborhood again," and "Cancer brought me closer to my husband and children." Thriving also can involve survivors reaching out to support others and to give back something tangible for all the care they received (Leight, 1998).

The best way to encourage thriving is to coach survivors in living each moment to the fullest and to find positive growth in the process and art of surviving (Dow, 1990).

The most visible creators I know of are those artists whose medium is life itself. The ones who express the inexpressible—without brush, hammer, clay or guitar. They neither paint nor sculpt—their medium is being. Whatever their presence touches has increased life. They see and don't have to draw. They are the artists of being alive. (Author Unknown)

REFERENCES

Abbey, M. (1997). Surviving cancer: A review of the impact and consequences. *Nursing Standard, 12*(4), 44–47.

Abrams, R. & Finesigner, J.L. (1953). Guilt reactions in patients with cancer. *Cancer, 6,* 474–482.

Ader, R., Madden, K., Felten, D.L., Bellinger, D.L. & Schiffer, R.B. (1996). Psychoneuroimmunology: Interactions between the brain and the immune system. In B.S. Fogel, R.B. Schiffer, & S.M. Rao (Eds.). *Neuropsychiatry.* Baltimore: Williams & Willkins.

Aguilera, D.C. (1994). *Crisis intervention: Theory and methodology.* St. Louis: Mosby.

American Cancer Society (1999). *Cancer facts and figures.* Atlanta, GA: Author.

American Psychiatric Association (1994). *Diagnostic and statistical manual of mental disorders* (4th ed.). Washington, D.C.: Author.

Anastasia, P.J. & Carroll-Johnson, R.M. (1998). Gender and age differences in the psychological response to cancer. In R.M. Carroll-Johnson, L.M. Gorman, & N.J. Bush (Eds.). *Psychosocial nursing care along the cancer continuum.* Pittsburgh: Oncology Nursing Press.

Archer-Copp, L. & Dixon-Copp, J. (1993). Illness and the human spirit. *Quality of Life: A Nursing Challenge: Spiritual Well-Being, 2(3),* 50–55.

Bard, M. & Dyk, R. (1956). The psychodynamic significance of beliefs regarding the cause of serious illness. *Psychoanalytic Review, 43,* 143–162.

Beyer, D.A. (1995). Cancer is a chronic disease. *Nurse Practitioner Forum, 6*(4), 201–206.

Breaden, K. (1997). Cancer and beyond: The question of survivorship. *Journal of Advanced Nursing, 26,* 978–984.

Bushkin, E. (1995). Signposts of survivorship. *Oncology Nursing Forum, 16,* 435–437.

Carter, B.J. (1989). Cancer survivorship: A topic for nursing research. *Oncology Nursing Forum, 16,* 435–437.

Cella, D.F., Mahon, S.M. & Donovan, M.I. (1990). Cancer recurrence as a traumatic event. *Behavioral Medicine, 16*(1), 15–22.

Clark, E.J. & Stovall, E.L. (1996). Advocacy: The cornerstone of cancer survivorship. *Cancer Practice, 4*(5), 239–244.

Cohen, F. & Lazarus, R.S. (1983). Coping and adaptation in health and illness. In D. Mechanic (Ed.). *Handbook of health: Health care and the health professions.* New York: Free Press.

Crothers, H. (1987). Health insurance: Problems and solutions for people with cancer histories. *Proceedings of the 5th National Conference on Human Values and Cancer.* San Francisco, CA: American Cancer Society.

Daum, A. & Collins, C. (1992). Failure to master early developmental tasks as a predictor of adaptation to cancer in the young adult. *Oncology Nursing Forum, 19*, 1513–1518.

Davies, R.K., Quinlan, D.M., McKegney, F.P. & Kimball, C.P. (1973). Organic factors and psychological adjustment in advanced cancer patients. *Psychosomatic Medicine, 35(6)*, 464–471.

Dow, K.H. (1990). The enduring seasons of survival. *Oncology Nursing Forum, 17*, 511–516.

Dow, K.H., Ferrell, B.R. & Anello, C. (1997). Balancing demands of cancer surveillance among survivors of thyroid cancer. *Cancer Practice, 5(5)*, 289–295.

Erikson, E.H. (1963). *Childhood and society*. New York: W.W. Norton.

Fehring, R.J., Miller, J.F., & Shaw, C. (1997). Spiritual well-being, religiosity, hope, depression, and other mood states in elderly people coping with cancer. *Oncology Nursing Forum, 24(4)*, 663–678.

Feldman, F.L. (1987). Female cancer patients and caregivers: Experiences in the workplace. In S. Stellamn (Ed.). *Women and cancer*. New York: Haworth Press.

Ferrell, B.R. & Dow, K.H. (1996). Portraits of cancer survivorship. *Cancer Practice, 4(2)*, 76–80.

Ferrel, B.R., Dow, K.H., Leigh, S., Ly, J., & Gulasekaram, P. (1995). Quality of life in long-term cancer survivors. *Oncology Nursing Forum, 22(6)*, 915–922.

Ferrell, B.R., Grant, M., Padilla, G., et al. (1991). The experience of pain and perceptions of quality of life: Validation of a conceptual model. *Hospice Journal, 7(3)*, 9–24.

Fiore, N.A. (1979). Fighting cancer: One patient's perspective. *New England Journal of Medicine, 300*, 284–289.

Fleck, A.E. (1993). Cancer economics. In S.L. Groenwald, M.H. Frogge, M. Goodman, & C.H. Yarbro (Eds.). *Cancer nursing: Principles and practice*. Boston: Jones & Bartlett.

Folkman, S. & Lazarus, R.S. (1980). An analysis of coping in a middle-aged community sample. *Journal of Health and Social Behavior, 21*, 219–239.

Frankl, V. (1959). *Man's search for meaning*. New York: Simon & Schuster.

Gorman, L. (1998). The psychosocial impact of cancer on the individual, family, and society. In R. Carroll-Johnson, L. Gorman, & M.J. Bush (Eds) *Psychosocial nursing along the cancer care continuum*. Pittsburgh: Oncology Nursing Press.

Gotay, S. (1985). Why me? Attributions and adjustment by cancer patients and their mates at two stages in the disease process. *Social Science Medicine, 20*, 825–831.

Haberman, M. (1996). Suffering and survivorship. In B.R. Ferrell (Ed.). *Suffering*. Boston: Jones & Barlett.

Halstead, M.T. & Fernsler, J.I. (1994). Coping strategies of long-term cancer survivors. *Cancer Nursing, 17(2)*, 94–100.

Hawkins, M.M. & Stevens, M.C.G. (1996). The long-term survivors. *British Medical Bulletin, 52(4)*, 898–923.

Hickey, S. (1986). Enabling hope. *Cancer Nursing, 9*, 133–137.

Hoffman, B. (1989). Cancer survivors at work: Job problems and illegal discrimination. *Oncology Nursing Forum 16(1)*, 39–43.

Hoffman, B. (1990). Taking care of business: Employment, insurance, and money matters. In F. Mullan & B. Hoffman (Eds.) *Charting the journey: An almanac of practical resources for cancer survivors*. Mount Vernon, NY: Consumer Reports Books.

Hoffman, B. (1997). Is the Americans with Disabilities Act protecting cancer survivors from employment discrimination? *Cancer Practice, 5(2)*, 119–121.

Hollen, P.J. & Hobbie, W.L. (1995). Establishing comprehensive specialty follow-up clinics for long-term survivors of cancer: Providing systematic physiological and psychological support. *Support Care Cancer, 3*, 40–44.

Hulme, W.E. (1986). *Vintage years: Growing older with meaning and hope*. New York: Westminster Press.

Johnson, J. & Johnson, M.B. (1998). Programmatic approaches to psychosocial support. In R.M. Carroll-Johnson, L.M. Gorman, & N.J. Bush (Eds.). *Psychosocial nursing care along the cancer continuum*. Pittsburgh: Oncology Nursing Press.

Johnston-Taylor, E. (1993). The search for meaning among persons with cancer. *Quality of Life: A Nursing Challenge: Spiritual Well-Being, 2(3)*, 65–70.

Kobasa, S.C. (1979). Stressful life events, personality and health: An inquiry into hardiness. *Journal of Personality and Social Psychology, 37*, 1–11.

Kobasa, S.C. (1982). The hardy personality: Toward a social psychology of stress and health. In J. Suls & G. Sanders (Eds.). *Social psychology of health and illness*. Hillsdale, NJ: L. Erlbaum.

Koopmeiners, L., Post-White, J., Gutnecht, S., Ceransky, C., Nickelsen, K., Drew, D., Mackey, K.W., & Kreitzer, M.J. (1997). How healthcare professionals contribute to hope in patients with cancer. *Oncology Nursing Forum, 24(9)*, 1507–1513.

Lazarus, R.L. & Folkman, S. (1984). *Stress, appraisal and coping*. New York: Springer Publishing Company.

Lee, C.O. (1997). Quality of life and breast cancer survivors. Psychosocial and treatment issues. *Cancer Practice 5(5)*, 309–317.

Leigh, S. (1998). Survivorship. In C.C. Burke (Ed.). *Psychosocial dimensions of oncology nursing care*. Pittsburgh: Oncology Nursing Press.

Leigh, S., Boyle, D., Loescher, L.J., & Hoffman, B. (1993). Psychosocial issues of long-term survivors of adult cancer. In S.L. Groenwald, M.H. Frogge, M. Goodman, & C.H. Yarbro (Eds.). *Cancer nursing: Principles and practice* (3rd ed.). Boston: Jones & Bartlett.

Loescher, L.J., Clark, L., Atwood, J.R. (1990). The impact of the cancer experience on long-term survivors. *Oncology Nursing Forum, 17*, 223–229.

Loney, M. (1999). Loss, grief, and dying. In W.J. Phipps, J.K. Sands, & J.F. Marek (Eds.). *Medical surgical nursing* (6th ed.). St. Louis: Mosby.

Mages, N.L., & Mendelsohn, G.A. (1980). Effects of cancer on patients' lives: A personological approach. In G.C. Stone, F. Cohen, & N.E. Adler (Eds.). *Health psychology: A handbook*. San Francisco: Jossey-Bass.

McCaffery, M. & Beebe, A. (1989). *Pain: A clinical manual for nursing practice*. St. Louis: Mosby.

Miller, J.F. (1985). Assessment of loneliness and spiritual well-being in chronically ill and healthy adults. *Journal of Professional Nursing, 1(2)*, 45–49.

Miller, J.F. (1992). *Coping with chronic illness: Overcoming powerlessness*. Philadelphia: F.A. Davis.

Moberg, D.O. (1980). Social indicators of spiritual well-being. In J.A. Thorson & T.C. Cook (Eds.). *Spiritual well-being of the elderly*. Springfield, IL: Charles C. Thomas.

Mullan, R. (1984). Re-entry: The educational needs of the cancer survivor. *Health Education Quarterly, 10*(Suppl.), 88–94.

Mullan, F. (1985). Seasons of survival: Reflections of a physician with cancer. *New England Journal of Medicine, 313*, 270–273.

O'Conner, A.P., Wicker, C.A., & Germino, B.B. (1990). Understanding the cancer patient's search for meaning. *Cancer Nursing, 13*, 167–175.

Osterman, P. & Schwartz-Barcott, D. (1996). Presence: Four ways of being there. *Nursing Forum, 31*(2), 23–30.

Ostchega, Y. & Jacob, J.G. (1984). Providing "safe conduct": Helping your patient cope with cancer. *Nursing 84, 34*(4), 42–47.

Padilla, G.V., Ferrell, B., Grant, M.M., et al. (1990). Defining the content domain of quality of life for cancer patients with pain. *Cancer Nurse, 13*(2), 108–115.

Pellegrino, D. (1982). Being ill and being healed. In V. Kestenbaum (Ed.). *Humanity of the ill: Phenomenological perspectives*. Knoxville: University of Tennessee Press.

Pelusi, J. (1997). The lived experience of surviving breast cancer. *Oncology Nursing Forum, 24*(4), 1343–1353.

Predeger, E. (1996). Womanspirit: A journey into healing through art in breast cancer. *Advances in Nursing Science, 18*(3), 48–58.

Raines, M.L. (1998). Problems with social support. In R.M. Carroll-Johnson, L.M. Gorman, & N.J. Bush (Eds.). *Psychosocial nursing care along the cancer continuum*. Pittsburgh: Oncology Nursing Press.

Rendle, K. (1997). Survivorship and breast cancer: The psychosocial issues. *Journal of Clinical Nursing, 6*, 403–410.

Rickel, L.M. (1987). Making mountains manageable: Maximizing quality of life through crisis intervention. *Oncology Nursing Forum, 14*, 28–34.

Scott, D.W., Donahue, D.C., Mastrovito, R.C., & Hakes, T.B. (1986). Comparative trial of clinical relaxation and an antiemetic drug and vomiting. *Cancer Nursing, 9*, 178–187.

Shanfield, S. (1980). On surviving cancer: Some psychological considerations. *Comprehensive Psychiatry, 21*(2), 128–134.

Spiegel, D. (1993). *Living beyond limits: New hope and help for facing life-threatening illness*. New York: Times Books.

Stuber, M.L., Kazak, A.E., Meeske, K., Barakat, L., Gurthrie, D., Garnier, H., Pynoos, R., & Meadows, A. (1997). Predictors of posttraumatic stress symptoms in childhood cancer survivors. *Pediatrics, 100*(6), 958–964.

Taylor, S. (1983). Adjustment to threatening events. *American Psychologist, 38*(11), 1161–1173.

Taylor, S., Lichtman, R. & Wood, J. (1984). Attributions, beliefs about control and adjustment to breast cancer. *Journal of Personality and Social Psychology, 46*(3), 489–502.

Tuls-Halstead, M. & Fernsler, J.I. (1994). Coping strategies of long-term cancer survivors. *Cancer Nursing, 17*(2), 94–100.

Van der Pompe, G., Antoni, M.H., Mulder, C.L., Heijnen, C., Goodkin, K., De Graeff, A., Garssen, B. & De Vries, M.J. (1994). Psychoneuroimmunology and the course of breast cancer: An overview. *Psycho-oncology, 3*(4), 271–288.

Van Fleet, S.K. (1998). Crisis intervention. In R.M. Carroll-Johnson, L.M. Gorman, & N.J. Bush (Eds.). *Psychosocial nursing care along the cancer continuum*. Pittsburgh: Oncology Nursing Press.

Varricchio, C. (1987). Cultural and ethnic dimensions of cancer nursing care: Introduction. *Oncology Nursing Forum, 14*(3), 57–58.

Wallace, K.G. (1997). Analysis of recent literature concerning relaxation and imagery interventions for cancer pain. *Cancer Nursing, 20*(2), 79–87.

Weekes, D. (1998). Cultural influences on the psychosocial experience. In R.M. Carroll-Johnson, L.M. Gorman, & N.J. Bush (Eds.). *Psychosocial nursing care along the cancer continuum*. Pittsburgh: Oncology Nursing Press.

Weisman, A. (1979). *Coping with cancer*. New York: McGraw-Hill.

Epidemiology of Cancer

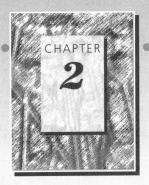

CHAPTER 2

Wende Levy

Epidemiology is the study of the distribution and determinants of disease in a population. Cancer is not considered an epidemic disease, but the principles of epidemiology are used to study cancer. Epidemiology is used in cancer care to improve the definition and classification of cancers. This approach also assists in the identification of factors leading to the development of cancer.

Cancer is the second leading cause of death in the United States. Twelve million new cases have been diagnosed since 1990. The American Cancer Society has stated that more than 1500 people are expected to die each day from cancer (Landis, Murray, Bolden, & Wingo, 1998). In 1996, cancer contributed to 23.3% of all deaths in the United States, yet overall 5-year survival rates have improved for most cancers, except for lung and bronchus (Figs. 2-1 and 2-2). In the next decade, our nation and healthcare systems will be challenged by the demand for resources to further reduce the incidence and mortality rates of this disease.

Prevention

The goal of epidemiologic studies and research is to prevent disease. Prevention comes from understanding the reasons for disease and the measures that can be taken to prevent them. Maintenance of health is a prime focus of epidemiology and is part of prevention and early detection of disease. There are currently three levels of prevention: primary, secondary, and tertiary (Johnson, 1994).

Primary prevention is the ability to avoid or eliminate the causative agent. Secondary prevention is strongly tied to early detection and treatment, such as in breast cancer. Tertiary treatment involves treatment of the cancer and symptom management. The focus of epidemiology studies in recent years has been on primary prevention. Many examples of these findings are seen every day. One example is the multiplicity of medicinal, marketing, and behavioral strategies being developed to assist people to avoid cigarettes and nicotine. Another is the education of the population regarding the outcomes from prolonged exposure to the sun and sunburns at an early age. Understanding the causes of cancer allows physicians and health care providers to screen individuals for cancer, educate them about the causes of cancer, and prevent certain cancers by early intervention. In general, early intervention in cancer treatment can decrease both the morbidity and mortality of cancer, but this is not always the case.

Studies on the epidemiology of cancer are designed to assess individual risk of developing cancer and identify the causes of cancer. Prevention strategies utilize this information to target individuals and specific populations for education and early intervention. In studies, the relative risk is a measure of the relationship between the cancer and the risk factors. For example, the American Cancer Society states that smokers have a ten-fold relative risk of developing lung cancer compared with nonsmokers. Risk is also described in terms of lifetime risk (American Cancer Society website, *http://www.cancer.org/statistics/cff99*, 1999).

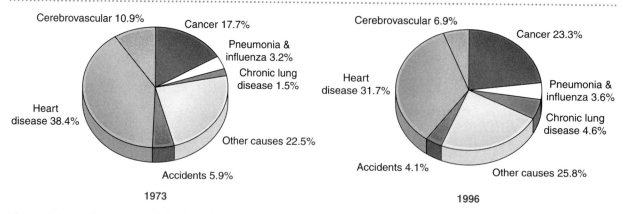

Figure 2-1 Leading causes of death in the U.S.: Percent of all causes of death, 1973 vs. 1996.

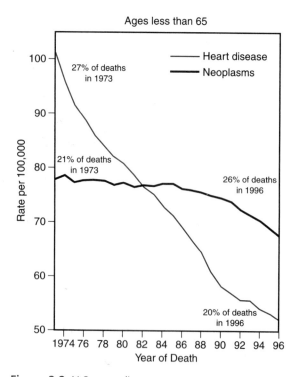

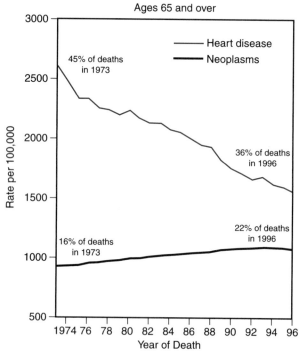

Figure 2-2 U.S. mortality rates, 1973 to 1996.